Pains *and* Planes

A Doctor's COVID-19 Memoir

VICTOR G. VOGEL, MD

Pains and Planes: A Doctor's COVID-19 Memoir
Copyright © 2025 by Victor G. Vogel, MD

ISBN: 979-8894790909(sc)
ISBN: 979-8894790916(e)

The Reading Glass Books
(888) 420-3050
www.readingglassbooks.com
fulfillment@readingglassbooks.com

Acknowledgement

The quoted Bible verses are from the
Holy Bible, New International Version,
Zondervan, Grand Rapids, Michigan, 2002.

Pains and Planes:
A Doctor's COVID-19 Memoir

This book is based on a diary kept by the author in the early months of 2021 at the onset of the COVID-19 pandemic. He was a full-time medical oncologist at the time, taking care of hundreds of women with breast cancer. As a general aviation pilot for 40 years and anticipating retirement from medicine, he also founded in late 2020 an educational public charity called **Susquehanna STEM to the Skies,** a 501(c)(3) registered with both the IRS and the PA Department of State and based at the Penn Valley Airport in Selinsgrove, Pennsylvania. It seeks to develop STEM (Science, Technology, Engineering, and Mathematics) educational opportunities in local schools with an aviation focus to help broaden school-based STEM education. It alerts students and teachers to the myriad employment opportunities within the aviation field, including pilots, mechanics, air traffic controllers, airport managers, airline dispatchers, and drone operators.

The COVID-19 pandemic caused severe social and economic disruption worldwide, including the most extensive global recession since the Great Depression. Widespread supply shortages, including food shortages, were caused by supply chain disruptions and panic buying. Reduced human activity led to an unprecedented temporary decrease in pollution. Many jurisdictions partially or fully closed educational institutions and public areas, and many events were canceled or postponed during 2020 and 2021. Telework became much more common for white-collar workers as the pandemic evolved. Misinformation circulated through social media and mass media, and political tensions intensified. The pandemic raised issues of racial and geographic discrimination, health equity, and the balance between public health imperatives and individual rights.

The US recorded 31.8 million new COVID-19 cases in 2021, up 59% from just under 20 million in 2020. Two states had a lower case count in 2021 than in 2020: North Dakota and South Dakota. Hawaii had the lowest case rate, with 6% of its population testing positive, while West Virginia had the highest, at 14%.

Non-Hispanic white people accounted for 65% of COVID-19 deaths in 2021 while making up slightly less than 60% of the US population. That gap is the biggest among seven racial and ethnic groups for which the CDC has data available. The other groups with more COVID-19 deaths relative to their population were three non-Hispanic groups: Black, American Indian or Alaska Native, and Native Hawaiian or Pacific Islander.

As of December 29, **456,789 deaths in 2021** were attributed to COVID-19, up 29% from 355,294 deaths in 2020. The rise in fatalities was not uniform across the country. While the number of deaths in 2021 more than doubled in 15 states over the previous year, deaths decreased in 12 states and Washington, DC. States hit hard in 2020 — Connecticut, New Jersey, New York, North Dakota, and Massachusetts — all had more than 40% fewer COVID-19 deaths in 2021.

Source of COVID-19 data: USAFacts.org is a not-for-profit, nonpartisan civic initiative making government data accessible for all.

KAIROS

In ancient Greek, *kairos* means "time," not just any time (Baert, 2020). It is about timeliness, the special moment when it's the opportune time to say or do something. Modern rhetoric refers to making the right statement at the right moment. In modern Greek, *kairos* also means 'weather' (Baert, 2020). It is one of two words the ancient Greeks had for 'time'; the other is *chronos*. Whereas the latter refers to chronological or sequential time, *kairos* signifies a proper or opportune time for action. The author used the Daily *Kairos* diary to record his thoughts during the pandemic.[1]

Each daily entry consists of a Bible passage from the New International Version translation, a statement of gratitude for the blessings I have received, a short prayer of concern for patients, coworkers, friends, and family, a plan for the day, and a record of what I was doing that day in my life and medical practice. Each day also contains a statement about what I will strive to do or become that day.

---

1 Kairos: The right moment or occasion. (2020, June 30). Institute for Advanced Study. *https://www.ias.edu/ideas/baert-kairos*

About the Author

D
r. Victor Vogel became a private pilot in 1980 and has flown more than 45 years with more than 2600 hours of flying experience. He became a certificated flight instructor (CFI) in 2019 and an instrument instructor in 2020. He has owned a Cirrus SR22 (N625VS) for 19 years. He is a retired medical oncologist with 36 years of experience doing clinical research in breast cancer. He was Professor of Medicine and Epidemiology at the University of Pittsburgh School of Medicine and National Vice President for Research for the American Cancer Society. He is an FAA Safety Team Representative for the Harrisburg, PA Flight Standards District Office. He is a member of the Board of Directors of the National Association of Flight Instructors (NAFI). He is the founder and president of Susquehanna STEM to the Skies, an educational public charity [501 (c) (3)] that introduces high school and technical center youth to aviation career opportunities. He has a special interest in the physiological effects of aging on flight safety.

Introduction

I picked up this journal as a gift from Seth Ziegler at our Thursday morning men's Bible study.

Building a habit of nurturing my relationship with God is important because, without God, I can do nothing. He has great plans for me, and I want to discern his will for my remaining life.

When I worked to build this habit, I struggled because other things constantly intruded and demanded my time.

I pledged that during the ensuing three months, I was going to do the following to help me stay focused:

1. Read the Bible each day.

2. Praise specifically for those I love and for what I need.

3. Seek to discern God's will for my life.

4. Confess my sins and seek God's forgiveness.

I was not going to expect perfection from myself. Instead, my goal was to seek the perfection in God and his creation and do what I can with what I have where I am.

THE DAILY KAIROS

Day 1, Isaiah 40: 30-31

> Even youths grow tired and weary,
> and young men stumble and fall;
> but those who hope in the Lord
> will renew their strength.
>
> They will soar on wings like eagles;
> They will run and not grow weary,
> they will walk and not be faint.

Gratitude

1. Sally, my wife, our children, and grandchildren
2. My professional life in medicine and the opportunity to contribute to knowledge that will end the suffering of women with breast cancer

Prayer

> Lord, make me rely not on my strength and understanding but on your truth so that I may rise up on eagles' wings and meet the needs of your people.

Today I will trust in the Lord with all my heart.

What I was doing on this day

I was preparing to lead today's Engaging Scripture class to read Isaiah 40 and 1 Corinthians 9. My wife Sally helped with the study. The apostle Paul admonished the Corinthians to surrender their freedom to sin and seek God's will to receive their spiritual renewal and liberation. I was greatly aided by Roger Gench in *Presbyterian Outlook* and his commentary on Isaiah 40.

Pilot and certificated flight instructor Chantelle Puletasi was sent to help Susquehanna STEM to the Skies. Dean Moyer and Russ Stankiewicz offered financial help to purchase a Cirrus SR22 panel for the Redbird FMX simulator.

Day 2, Psalm 25: 14

> The LORD confides in those who fear him; he makes his covenant known to them.

> I am thankful for Dr. Gene Heid, Yvonne Dansoa, and Penn Valley Airport. I also thank God for Bill and Kristen Morrow, who came to watch Super Bowl LV.

Prayer

> Lord, bring healing to (patient name) and heal her fractured tibial plateau. And bring peace and healing to (patient name) with his locally advanced small-cell lung cancer. God bless Gene Heid, who is becoming a personal friend. I called Gene, and he spoke to me about Laurie Garrett, her book *The Coming Plague*, and his patient at York Hospital, who had Lassa fever.

> I will seek the Lord's will for my life.

What I was doing on this day

I am troubled by those patients who have lost their faith in medicine and in physicians who think they can research the proper treatment for their breast cancer. But whom do they read? Who are the authorities they seek? Why do answers on the Internet have more credibility than the recommendations of a physician?

Day 3, Jeremiah: 3: 19

"I myself said,

'How gladly would I treat you like my children and give you a pleasant land, the most beautiful inheritance of any nation.'
I thought you would call me 'Father' and not turn away from following me."

Gratitude

1. My wife, Sally
2. 7 grandchildren
3. Susquehanna STEM to the Skies

Lord, please grant insight and peace, acceptance, and gratitude to <Dr. Colleague>. Teach him to listen and to try to understand others. Show him the value of palliative care and hospice. And cause me to be more patient with him.

Prayer

Today, I will share the hope of the Gospel with <Dr. Colleague> (I never was able to do this).

What I was doing on this day

I was caring for the sick. There was a prisoner from the Muncie women's prison with a 19-centimeter cancer in her left breast. She had large, palpable left axillary lymph nodes and a posterior left cervical node. A patient of mine from Africa asked for the COVID-19 vaccine. Another patient had right axillary and subclavian thrombosis. A colleague was obsessed with the second impeachment trial of President Trump. I contacted an insurance company to get a liability quote for the Redbird FMX simulator.

I bought ice melt at Cole's Hardware and Honey Nut Cheerios at Dollar General. Christie Gower was a blessing today.

Day 4, Revelation 4: 11

> "You are worthy, our Lord and God,
> to receive glory and honor and power,
> For you created all things,
> and by your will they were created
> and have their being."

Gratitude

1. Sally, Heather, and Christiaan
2. My profession and the trainees
3. My aviation avocation
4. School board member Virginia Zimmerman called with the names of the Lewisburg area school district Superintendent and high school principal.

A prayer for healing for three patients and a colleague.

What I was doing on this day

I taught a second-year internal medicine resident the fundamentals of breast cancer for a primary care physician. I saw and treated 12 patients. I prepared a lesson for the Penn Valley Pilots about in-flight icing and its risks. Chantelle Puletasi scheduled a meeting with Midd-West High School about STEM curriculum. I made consult rounds in the hospital.

I saw God in the person of an interested and committed second-year resident and in a first-year fellow who is showing continued improvement in his medical oncology skills.

Day 5, Psalm 19: 14

> May these words of my mouth and this meditation of my heart be pleasing in your sight, Lord, my Rock, and my Redeemer. (remembering my father, a pastor, who always prayed this prayer before delivering a sermon)

Gratitude

1. Men's Bible study
2. A colleague with a fracture who does not need a knee replacement
3. Patients who are well (a young woman with triple-negative breast cancer had a negative PET/CT scan following preoperative chemotherapy)

Prayer

> Lord, grant peace to my patient with a new diagnosis of metastatic breast cancer. Please help us to find an effective, non-toxic treatment. Make the latest member of our Bible study one of us and open our hearts to his presence.

Today, I will trust in the Lord to bring peace and healing to patients when I cannot.

What I was doing on this day

God caused my colleague to be silent at times today. Christie Gower was a tremendous administrative help. Jennie Reinard is a fabulous nurse. Charity Miller, LPN, is a constant help. I bought Valentine's flowers for Sally three days early so she could enjoy them.

I am grateful that two patients have completed seven years of aromatase inhibitor therapy.

Day 6, Hebrews 11:16

> Instead, they were longing for a better country—a heavenly one. Therefore, God is not ashamed to be called their God, for he has prepared a city for them.

Gratitude

1. My back was pain-free this morning.
2. For Susquehanna STEM to the Skies
3. For Larry Bonner (physician assistant) and Jasmine Martin (hematology/oncology fellow)
4. For our excellent hematology/oncology fellows

Prayer

> Relieve Dale's back pain and Seth's chest pain. Comfort HA in her distress and give her peace in her crisis— Grant DS success in his quest. Open our minds to those who are different.

Today, I told myself I would rejoice in being the late doctor in the clinic.

What I was doing on this day

Again, I enjoyed teaching a second-year medical resident about breast cancer and doing consultations with one of our medical oncology fellows. I enjoyed seeing my patient with schizophrenia. I also enjoyed watching the aviation program *AOPA Live*. I wrestled with setting up my new laptop. I watched *The Affair* on Prime Video.

God was present today in the intensive care unit with us, and a young man recently diagnosed with locally advanced small-cell lung cancer is about to begin chemotherapy.

Day 7, Proverbs 19: 17

> Whoever is kind to the poor lends to the Lord, and he will reward them for what they have done.

Gratitude

1. Sally and the children
2. Flying and being a CFI
3. Being an airplane owner
4. Susquehanna STEM to the Skies

Prayer

> Grant safety to my student pilot through an understanding of the responsibilities of a pilot to maintain safety. Give him an understanding and clarity that will keep him and others safe.

Today, I will acknowledge my imperfections and trust in the Lord.

What I was doing on this day

My student forgot to remove the tow bar from the nose gear of the airplane, and we had a prop strike with the tow bar attached. I neglected to assure him that he had removed the bar. I flew with Brady Fries in N625VS, and we both greased our landings. I flew the inaugural instructional flight for currency in the Redbird FMX with Garrett Hupp. I met a dentist from Kenya who works in Selinsgrove and is interested in learning to fly.

Day 8, St. Valentine's Day, I Corinthians 13: 4-7

> Love is patient; love is kind. It does not envy, it does not boast, it is not proud. It does not dishonor others, it is not self-seeking, it is not easily angered, it keeps no record of wrongs. Love does not delight in evil but rejoices with the truth. It always protects, always trusts, always hopes, always perseveres.

Gratitude

1. For Sally's love for more than 46 years.
2. For the First Presbyterian Church, Lewisburg
3. For the Engaging Scripture Bible study and for Bonnie Troxell

Prayer

> Lord, give us Christians strength in these trying times. Help us remember the courage and faith of those before us.

Today, I will rest, relax, and trust in the Lord. I will celebrate Sally and our marriage.

What I was doing on this day

Our Engaging Scripture class today studied the transfiguration in Mark 4 and 1 Corinthians 4, Paul's warning to the Christians of Corinth to be different than those with whom they lived. Ryan Krause's sermon was a warning to "Follow me." Sally and I enjoyed an excellent Sunday dinner, and Sally made Valentine's heart cookies and took them to Bible study class members. There was an installation of elders, deacons, and trustees at the church. I enjoyed an afternoon of peaceful rest. Sally and I exchanged Valentine's gifts.

Day 9, 2 Corinthians 4: 1- 6

> Therefore, since through God's mercy we have this ministry, we do not lose heart. Instead, we have renounced secret and shameful ways; we do not use deception or distort the word of God. On the contrary, by setting forth the truth plainly we commend ourselves to everyone's conscience in the sight of God. And even if our gospel is veiled, it is veiled to those who are perishing. The god of this age has blinded the minds of unbelievers so that they cannot see the light of the gospel that displays the glory of Christ, who is the image of God. For what we preach is not ourselves, but Jesus Christ as Lord, and ourselves as your servants for Jesus' sake. For God, who said, "Let light shine out of darkness," and make his light shine in our hearts to give us the light of the knowledge of God's glory displayed in the face of Christ.

Gratitude
1. For work
2. For Sally
3. For appreciative patients
4. For the smiles and laughter of our grandson Finnegan

Prayer

> Give comfort, courage, and peace to a friend who is
> entirely opposed to COVID-19 vaccination so that he
> might rejoin our Thursday Bible study. Bring healing
> for Dale and Seth and to our cousin, Dr. Phil Hacker,
> who was recently diagnosed with skin cancer.

Today, I will trust the Lord to lead my steps and guide my
thoughts.

What I was doing on this day

It was a delightful day in the clinic with a first-year fellow. Went
to the Breast Multidisciplinary Clinic with another first-year
fellow. We saw a 36-year-old woman with a 2-year-old son who
was leaving her husband. She had a 5-centimeter left breast
mass. She came to the clinic with her friend, who is a registered
nurse. There were many tears. We saw two consultations in
the hospital, including a prisoner on house arrest with lung
cancer as well as a kidney tumor. We also saw a young man
with a large retroperitoneal mass who was awaiting the results
of a needle biopsy. There was an ice storm in central PA, but
I could drive home without incident.

The Lord was in the room with us when we spoke to the
36-year-old woman and outlined our plans for her treatment,
which was to begin within the next ten days.

Day 10, Titus 3: 5

> He saved us not because of our righteous actions but
> because of his mercy. He saved us through the washing
> of rebirth and renewal by the Holy Spirit,

Gratitude

1. For learning to speak with Sally from my heart
2. For the friendship of Dr. Joseph Lynch
3. For the maturing competence of our second-year fellow

Prayer

For Paul Preidecker, Karen Kalishek, Bob Meder, Adam Magee, and all the members of the National Association of Flight Instructors (NAFI) board of directors and for the Session of the First Presbyterian Church of Lewisburg.

Today, I will listen more attentively during board and session meetings.

What I was doing on this day

Sometimes, God calls us to lay down our lives for him and the cause. More often, the Lord does not ask us to die for him. Instead, he calls us to live for him, a matter of lifelong service. Saint Paul said "I plead with you to give your bodies to God. Let them be a living and holy sacrifice he will accept." (Romans 12: 1)

God appeared today in the leadership of Paul Preidecker, President of NAFI. I am a member of their board of directors.

Day 11, Ash Wednesday, I John 4: 11-12

Dear friends, since God loved us so much, we should also love one another. No one has ever seen God, but if we love one another, God lives in us, and his love is made complete in us.

Gratitude

For the life of Rush Limbaugh, who died today at the age of 70 from lung cancer. Serena Tripp, Rosemary Leeming, Nicole Deckard, and Julie Hergenrather each serve women well in our cancer genetics clinics.

Prayer

For Katherine Limbaugh and our country. For the political left, who will castigate Mr. Limbaugh even after his death. For a dear patient with progressive disease, that our treatment will be both effective and helpful.

Today, I will be more mindful of patients who live with uncertainty about their medical futures.

What I was doing on this day

We saw 12 patients in the breast clinic this morning, and our resident and fellow did an admirable job, for which I am thankful. We saw four new patients with CDH1, BRCA1/2, and CHEK2 mutations in the breast cancer genetics clinic. I pray that the women with the *CHEK2* mutation do not develop gastric cancer, which is not common with that mutation but can occur. Sally and I watched *The Affair*, which confirms that adultery is a very messy situation. One of my colleagues did hospital consultations so that I did not have to do them. I gave Dr. Joseph Lynch an autographed copy of the article I wrote in 1987 with Rick Jones on veno-occlusive disease of the liver.

Day 12, I John 4: 17

This is how love is made complete among us so we

will have confidence on the day of judgment: In this world, we are like Jesus.

Gratitude

My physician colleague took the day off, and the silence was golden. Our morning Bible study was true fellowship. Bill Morrow gave me the name of a parent from the Columbia County Christian School who expressed interest in our STEM program, and for the Bach Choir of Bethlehem, Pennsylvania.

Prayer

That two colleagues would accept one another and be welcomed into our Bible study group. I pray for healing for a patient with brain metastases and two others with progressive breast cancer on the skin of their chests.

What I was doing on this day

Today, I will know that God will grant me the strength to accomplish all my tasks. I was thinking about Ryan Farran, a missionary Bush pilot in Papua New Guinea, and I pray for his mission and safety. I was concerned about how I would manage the time demands of our STEM program, writing, teaching two Bible studies, and teaching our fellows.

I celebrated receiving a galley proof of my article on fatigue in pilots from Frank Bowlin, editor of *IFR Magazine*.

There is less snow than forecast.

Day 13, Psalm 119:26

I gave an account of my ways, and you answered me; teach me your decrees.

Gratitude

Sally, Heather, and Christiaan, and for health. Our grandchildren, my Cirrus airplane, and Susquehanna STEM to the Skies. Chantelle Puletasi, Brady Fries, Walter Okumu.

Prayer

For health care for Judy Dillon in Texas and Dr. Phil Hacker in Wisconsin. For Liza and Jim Glenney and their daughters. For Cheryl and Johnny Burns, for Seth Ziegler, and Dale Lind.

Today, I will visit Midd-West High School to promote their STEM program.

What I was doing on this day

I was speaking with a 31-year-old man about his unresectable, metastatic, retroperitoneal sarcoma with one of our medical oncology fellows and a physician assistant. God was with us in that room. I also had a long conversation with the mother of a 10th grader in the Civil Air Patrol squadron at Bloomsburg Airport. His physics teacher is interested in promoting a STEM program in their high school.

Day 14, Colossians 3: 17

And whatever you do, whether in word or deed, do it all in the name of the Lord Jesus, giving thanks to God the Father through him.

Gratitude

The Philmont Scout Ranch grace:

For food, for raiment,
For life, for opportunity,
For friendship and fellowship,
We thank thee, O Lord. Amen

Prayer

For Lewisburg, Midd-West, and Columbia County Christian high schools. For Sally's drive to Pittsburgh tomorrow.

Today, I will not lean to my understanding but, in all my ways, acknowledge him.

What I was doing on this day

I spent 1.7 hours in the Redbird FMX simulator at the airport. I put high-visibility tape on the floor and hung the framed letter from the FAA indicating that we have an approved advanced aviation training device, an AATD. I sent an e-mail to the board of directors of Susquehanna STEM to the Skies advising them and updating them on our progress. Sally helped me with my work at the simulator.

Day 15, the First Sunday in Lent, Psalm 25: 1-2, 4, 7

In you, Lord my God, I put my trust.
I trust in you; do not let me be put to shame,
nor let my enemies triumph over me.
Show me your ways, Lord, teach me your paths.
Do not remember the sins of my youth and my rebellious ways; remember me according to your love, for you, Lord, are good.

Gratitude

For the burden of opportunity and the gift of talent and ability. For Dr. Russell Stankiewicz and the members of the board of directors of Susquehanna STEM to the Skies.

Prayer

Still my heart and let me know that you are the Lord. Teach me to love those who live in doubt and uncertainty and to show your courage to the afflicted. May I seek to love rather than to be loved, always remembering your grace and eternally guarding and comforting presence.

Today, I will not be afraid.

What I was doing on this day

The Engaging Scripture class had a good discussion about the Trinity. After putting ice melt on it yesterday, I drove to the airport and chipped ice in front of the hangar. I emptied the Cirrus for its upcoming annual inspection, updated the databases, and used the Best Tug to move the plane out of the hangar. I put my car in the hangar. The ceiling and visibility were unlimited today, with the chilly outside temperature of 24 degrees without wind. I flew the Cirrus and did a chandelle and two lazy eights. I flew to Lancaster and flew the RNAV 26, RNAV 31, and VOR DME 8 approaches with a circle to land at Lancaster. I learned that the fixed base operator, Alliance, has moved to the terminal building. Russ Stankiewicz brought me home after I left the Cirrus at Lancaster for its annual inspection.

Catherine Pulsifer wrote, "Our prayers are sometimes answered without us realizing or, in ways that we did not ask for but always remember God's plan is better than ours."

Day 16, I John 2: 27

As for you, the anointing you received from him remains in you, and you do not need anyone to teach you. But as his anointing teaches you about all things and as that anointing is real, not counterfeit—just as it has taught you, remain in him.

Gratitude

I thank God for friends, health, Sally and family, work, avocation, and being a pilot and a teacher.

Prayer

Bring health and understanding to those I serve today. Keep my mind clear and my heart open to their distress. Grant me empathy and compassion. Bring healing to our patient with unresectable cancer and to all who are suffering.

Today, I will trust in the Lord.

What I was doing on this day

Our patients love our first-year fellow. We were displaced from the Orthopedics conference room at the Woodbine clinic. The Breast Multidisciplinary Clinic is a virtual event because of COVID-19. We see yet another woman younger than 50 years of age with triple negative breast cancer. Sally is in Pittsburgh getting Jessica and Christiaan's house ready for sale. God was present in our exam rooms today, primarily through our young medical oncology fellow. I fall asleep in front of the television.

Day 17, Proverbs 13: 12

Hope deferred makes the heart sick, but a longing fulfilled is a tree of life.

Gratitude

It was a light clinic day, and no one was terribly ill. Therefore, I had time to work on two PowerPoint slide presentations: one on spatial disorientation and the Kobe Bryant helicopter crash and another on checklists and standard operating procedures.

Prayer

I pray for those in my care, Sally's safe return, and Susquehanna STEM to the Skies.

Today, I trust that the STEM program will succeed.

What I was doing on this day

I answered questions for the IRS from our attorney, who is creating our 501 (c)(3) public charity. I sent Zoom meeting invitations to the leadership of Lewisburg High School. I am talking with our senior flight instructor, Dave Hall, about teaching in the Redbird FMX simulator.

Day 18, Acts 16:14

One of those listening was a woman from the city of Thyatira named Lydia, a dealer in purple cloth. She was a worshiper of God. The Lord opened her heart to respond to Paul's message.

Gratitude

For our hematology-oncology fellows, for my senior colleagues Joseph Lynch and Mellar Davis, for God at the bedside, and for a special patient who is dying.

Prayer

Guard Sally today in her travels. God bless flight instructor Max Trescott and his interest in Susquehanna STEM to the Skies.

Today, I will speak my mind with no regard for the criticism of others.

What I was doing on this day

I paid for the Redbird FMX replacement insurance online. We had an irritating staff meeting about global endocrine dysfunction with the checkpoint inhibitors. I feel that one of my colleagues does way too many laboratory tests during the post-treatment follow-up. One of my colleagues had difficulty understanding the limitations of our knowledge about coronavirus vaccines in patients receiving chemotherapy. One of my patients did not appreciate her treatment schedule, which I thought I had explained clearly.

God revealed himself today through Austin Oberholtzer, Jasmine Martin, and me as I examined a woman in her mid-50s with newly diagnosed lung metastases following a renal transplant.

Day 19, Mark 8:34.

Then he called the crowd to him, along with his disciples, and said, "Whoever wants to be my disciple must deny themselves, take up their cross, and follow me.

Gratitude

For the men in my Thursday morning Bible study. For Jenny Reinard, Joanne Serra, and all the treating nurses who care for my patients with love and professionalism.

Prayer

Grant healing to Seth Ziegler. Give Dean grace and courage to complete his ministry. Help Aunt Diane adjust to her new life as a widow.

Today, I will lead a prayerful and thoughtful Bible study on II Chronicles 7-11

What I was doing on this day

Tiffany Delp, RN, finished her chemo-immunotherapy today for her triple negative breast cancer. Her husband, a Lewisburg police officer, brought his colleagues, a fire truck, an ambulance, and a limousine to our clinic at 75 Medical Park Drive in Lewisburg. He was joined by nurses from the Evangelical Community Hospital, who clapped and cheered and set off confetti poppers when Tiffany left the clinic. It was the highlight of my week. We took pictures, and there was an article in the weekly community newspaper.

God is with me and those in my care.

Day 20, Luke 14:11

For all those who exalt themselves will be humbled, and those who humble themselves will be exalted."

Gratitude

For Todd Aungst, Dale Lind, Chantal Puletasi, and all who help with Susquehanna STEM to the Skies,

Sally, and my sister Louise. For my brother Tim and his wife Brenda. For Heather and Christiaan and the seven dwarfs, our grandchildren.

Prayer

Grant Russ and me clear thoughts and open minds, if it be your will, when we share our STEM vision with school leadership today. Grant that they will make STEM education a reality in the Lewisburg Area School District.

Today, I will speak clearly and humbly and trust God's presence in our Zoom meeting about STEM.

What I was doing on this day

We had a pleasant and optimistic Zoom meeting with the Lewisburg Area School District leadership. They expressed great interest in STEM education and the prospect of an aviation STEM activity club. I saw seven healthy follow-up patients in my morning clinic, and all were well. I discharged two of them from my care. I saw a new consultation with a primary lung cancer metastatic to her cerebellum. The prognosis is grave.

God was present in our Zoom calls. One of the fellows said that he could hear my voice when answering the breast cancer questions in the stage examination for the medical oncology board examination.

Day 21, Psalm 90:17

May the favor of the Lord our God rest on us;
establish the work of our hands for us—
Yes, establish the work of our hands.

Gratitude

For health, for Sally, our daughter Heather, our son Christiaan, and the Seven Dwarfs. For Fly Advanced for maintaining my Cirrus aircraft. For wealth and comfort. For opportunity and choices, which are tangible signs of wealth.

Prayer

Lord, teach me not to be anxious about the outcome of events in the future. Please help me learn to bear the burden of uncertainty in my life and in the lives of my patients.

Today, I will trust in the Lord and thank him for my manifold and countless blessings.

What I was doing on this day

I woke up at 5:00 AM and watched television. I worked on the lesson for the Engaging Scripture class, where we will study Mark 8: 31-38 and Psalm 22. The bill for the annual inspection for N625VS was $9200. I was troubled to learn that the computer in the room I called the Flight Deck would not turn on after downloading 23 driver updates. Sally and I fall asleep by 8:30 PM watching television. One of the fellows sent me a Tiger Text thanking me for preparing them to answer the breast cancer questions on the stage exam for the medical oncology board examination.

I am thankful for my job, my wife, my family, my health and wealth, comfort, friends, and opportunity, as well as the respect of my peers. I have much for which to be grateful.

Day 22, I Peter 3:12

For the eyes of the Lord are on the righteous.
And his ears are attentive to their prayer,
But the face of the Lord is against those who do evil.

Gratitude

For the Engaging Scripture class: David Shrom, Bonnie and John Troxell, Judith and Seth Ziegler, Amber Lind, Nancy Steckel, Glenn Dobbs, Sally, and Gene Heid.

Prayer

Grant Sally safe passage to Fairfax, Virginia. Give Heather peace of mind as she deals with the complexities of her move to Jacksonville. Bring healing to Seth Ziegler and comfort to Nancy and Glenn, both new widows, in their grief.

Today, I will dedicate myself to making the STEM project successful.

I taught the Engaging Scripture class on Mark 8:29 and the following, in which Peter declares, "You are the Christ!"

What I was doing on this day

I thought about taking up our crosses and following him. Our crosses are not our afflictions in suffering but our bearing the consequences of declaring the gospel and speaking out against social and political injustice. It is just 21 days until the spring equinox, and this long, trying winter ends. Reverend Ryan Krause's sermon spoke of our bearing our crosses for Christ's sake.

Day 23, Galatians 5:16-17

So, I say, walk by the Spirit, and you will not gratify the desires of the flesh. For the flesh desires what is contrary to the Spirit, and the Spirit what is contrary to the flesh. They are in conflict with each other so that you are not to do whatever you want.

Gratitude

For Yvonne Dansoa and Dan Carlson. For Larry Bonner.

Prayer

Grant peace and healing to all those in my care. Grant patience and understanding to Heather and peace to Tabitha and Tyson. Keep our son-in-law Stephen in your care. Make both Heather's and Christiaan's moves as smooth as possible.

Today, I will do less, trust more, and love the Lord.

What I was doing on this day

I reviewed a patient in the Breast Multidisciplinary Clinic who was told at a large Comprehensive Cancer Center to receive a specific therapy preoperatively. She subsequently had progression during the preoperative chemotherapy. We watched a presentation on labeled estradiol body imaging from a new company. I had thought of it at the University of Pittsburgh 20 years ago. Todd Adams from Lancaster Avionics said it would cost $7000 to fix my broken primary flight display. I am grateful that I have the resources to cover these repairs.

Day 24, Psalm 145:18-19

The Lord is near to all who call on him,
to all who call on him in truth.
He fulfills the desires of those who fear him;
he hears their cry and saves them.

Gratitude

I am thankful for my board of directors in the STEM program. They are excellent, dedicated, skillful people. I had a brief clinic day.

Prayer

Lord, help me in my loneliness and isolation. May I put my trust not in things but in you. Grant Heather peace in this time of transition.

Today, I told my colleague to stop perseverating about late-night calls with untimely laboratory data.

What I was doing on this day

We had a great meeting of the board of directors of Susquehanna STEM to the Skies. A sadness today was a 27-year-old with breast cancer who came to the clinic with her very understanding father.

Day 25, 1 Thessalonians 5:17

Pray continually.

Gratitude

For the growing maturity of Dr. Daniel Carlson. For solitude and rest and a break from duties and obligations.

Prayer

Bring Sally home safely and help her not to worry and obsess over details.

Today, I will believe that the STEM project will succeed

What I was doing on this day

I spoke with Glen Ponas at AOPA. Dale Lind had made the connection. Glen is the AOPA Director of the High School Outreach Program. He will help develop our liaison with the Central Susquehanna Intermediate Unit (CSIU) and the Lewisburg Area School District. For the first time, I am hopeful that we can make our STEM program successful. I did not need to see any new medical oncology consultations in the hospital today. Glen Ponas was the answer to an unstated but fervently felt prayer.

Day 26, Isaiah 49: 16

See, I have engraved you on the palms of my hands; your walls are ever before me.

Gratitude

For life, health, daily food, and solitude. For the people who maintain my Cirrus aircraft and its avionics. Bill Morrow led a great men's Bible study today. Both Bill Morrow and Dale Lind are blessings.

Prayer

Thanks for bringing Sally home safely after five days in Fairfax with Heather and the twins.

Today, I will not get angry at the expense of maintaining a personal airplane.

What I was doing on this day

I saw a 53-year-old woman with a 10-centimeter right breast cancer. She was a bodybuilder in the 1980s. I took the Flight Deck computer to Best Buy for repair. The operating system became corrupted after I installed 23 driver updates. Lancaster Avionics called to report a problem with my ADS-B transponder. It will cost $7000 to replace a blade in my Avidyne primary flight display. The "Foghorn" [my overly talkative colleague] was honking all day.

Day 27, Ephesians 3: 14-15

> For this reason, I kneel before the Father, from whom every family in heaven and on earth derives its name.

Gratitude

> I pray for Sally's safe arrival home, for all that I can accomplish and have the opportunity to do, and for those who helped me care for patients.

Prayer

> Grant relief, and if it be your will, cure to all those in my care.

Today, I will not be anxious about the future, knowing that they are in God's hands.

Day 28, Psalm 119: 25

> I am laid low in the dust; preserve my life according to your word.

Gratitude

> For Todd Aungst, our local FAA Designated Pilot

Examiner (DPE), I learned that he was an Eagle Scout. I spent one hour and 48 minutes in the Redbird FMX simulator, where I'm still learning my way around, for the promise of spring.

Prayer

Lord, calm my fears about the possible failures of Susquehanna STEM to the Skies. Lead me to trust in others and you.

Today, I will not be anxious about the future. Let go, let God.

What I was doing on this day

Todd Aungst spent an hour in the Redbird FMX. I taught him how to use the Navigator software on his iPad. He brought the replaced printer from his office and placed it on the desk in the simulator room. Sally drove to DuBois to see sister Peggy and her husband Tom. We had a spirited discussion on her return. We watched Liam Neeson's movie, *Honest Thief,* which was quite good.

God brought Todd Aungst into my STEM program. Things break (my flight deck computer) and either get fixed, or we move on.

Day 29, 1 John 4: 19-20

We love because he first loved us. Whoever claims to love God yet hates a brother or sister is a liar. For whoever does not love their brother and sister, whom they have seen, cannot love God, whom they have not seen.

Gratitude

For our Engaging Scripture class. For Bonnie Troxell. For glorious sunshine: Psalm 19:1 and John 2.

Prayer

Lead me to put my trust in you, oh Lord. Guide me to success, if it is your will, in the STEM to the Skies enterprise.

Today, I will relax and trust in the Lord.

What I was doing on this day

I am writing an abstract for the breast cancer webinar on March 17-18. I also need to record my presentation. I figured out how to do this with Zoom—record and the "share screen" feature. I had a 50-minute telephone conversation with Bonnie Troxell about the STEM program. She gave very helpful advice on identifying interested science teachers and riding their enthusiasm.

Day 30, 1 John 3: 14, Proverbs 4: 6-7

We know that we have passed from death to life because we love each other. Anyone who does not love remains in death.

Do not forsake wisdom, and she will protect you; love her, and she will watch over you.
The beginning of wisdom is this: Get wisdom.
Though it cost all you have, get understanding.

Gratitude

For patient JH, who had a complete pathological

response to a four-drug and immunological pre-operative therapy for her triple-negative breast cancer.

Thanks to those who serve our patients: the surgeons, the hematology/medical oncology fellows, the nurses, the pathologists, the secretaries, our social workers, our radiation oncologists, and our physician assistants. I am thankful for all of those who care for the sick and the dying.

Prayer

Lord, I want to know the secret to breast cancer. Show me its mysteries. Government money has not found the answer. Billions of commercial pharmaceutical dollars have not solved the problem. Make me faithful to your word and open my eyes to end the affliction. In Jesus name, Amen.

Today, I will be thankful for the healing we can bring.

Day 31, James 4:1-2

What causes fights and quarrels among you? Don't they come from your desires that battle within you? You desire but do not have, so you kill. You covet, but you cannot get what you want, so you quarrel and fight. You do not have because you do not ask God.

Gratitude

It was a short clinic day, a quiet Foghorn, a very competent nurse specialist, and an exceptionally beautiful late winter day. N625VS is back home in the hangar. When I departed Lancaster, I forgot to deploy the flaps before takeoff. Liftoff was predictably delayed but otherwise uneventful. I am thankful for nurses, airplane mechanics, and technicians who keep my patients and me safe.

Prayer

Lord, open my eyes that I might see. Reveal to me the mystery of breast cancer. Show me for the sake of the suffering and not for my reward. Do it soon, if it is your will. Stop the suffering. In his name. Amen.

Today, I will believe and see.

What I was doing on this day

I saw a very elderly and frail woman in the clinic following her admission for a stroke two weeks ago. We will stop her chemotherapy and give her a monoclonal antibody only for her stage 1 HER2-positive breast cancer.

I finished the clinic by 3:00 PM and went to the airport at 3:45 to meet Russ Stankiewicz, who flew me to Lancaster airport to pick up N625VS after its annual inspection. I talked with Russ and the mechanic on the ramp for 20 minutes in 65-degree weather. Spring has arrived.

Day 32, Psalm 145: 17

The Lord is righteous in all his ways and faithful in all he does.

Gratitude

My first-year fellow was very efficient in the clinic.

Prayer

Give me balance, Lord, with medicine, my flight instructor activities, and the STEM program.

Today, I will teach and heal with both compassion and gratitude.

What I was doing on this day

Sally drove to Elizabethtown because Christiaan and Jessica planned to buy their new home. We had an early dinner with Chris and the kids. I presented the NTSB/Paul Bertorelli review of the Kobe Bryant helicopter crash to the Penn Valley pilots, and I reviewed loss-of-control accidents and visual flight into instrument meteorological conditions. I did three full-stop landings in Cirrus N625VS. I got a "transponder unavailable" message when I exited the runway.

Day 33, Philippians 2: 14-15; Acts 2: 40, Ephesians 2: 1-3, Matthew 17: 17

> Do everything without grumbling or arguing so that you may become blameless and pure, "children of God without fault in a warped and crooked generation. Then you will shine among them like stars in the sky.

> With many other words he warned them; and he pleaded with them, "Save yourselves from this corrupt generation."

> As for you, you were dead in your transgressions and sins, in which you used to live when you followed the ways of this world and of the ruler of the kingdom of the air, the spirit who is now at work in those who are disobedient. All of us also lived among them at one time, gratifying the cravings of our flesh and following its desires and thoughts. Like the rest, we were by nature deserving of wrath.

"You unbelieving and perverse generation," Jesus replied, "how long shall I stay with you? How long shall I put up with you? Bring the boy here to me."

Gratitude

I went with Chris and the kids to Best Buy to pick up my Flight Deck computer and learned that it did not need an operating system reinstallation. The problem was CMOS, a depleted battery, and two viruses. My flight simulator program survived.

Prayer

Grant peace and clarity to our friend Dean, who has some odd ideas about your will. Show him that he is loved and help him realize your grace.

Today, I will thank the Lord for all his benefits.

What I was doing on this day

We had a marvelous Microsoft TEAMS meeting online with Glen Ponas, Carla Smith, and Colleen Epler-Ruths about the AOPA aviation STEM curriculum. Then, I got a call from a colleague at the Evangelical Community Hospital who said she was taking flying lessons and heard about the Redbird FMX simulator. She gave me the name of a flight instructor who is an Embry-Riddle Aviation University graduate who was asking questions about the FMX simulator. I then got a call from our senior flight instructor, who wanted to get checked out in the simulator.

Day 34, Psalm 107: 28-31

Then they cried out to the Lord in their trouble,
and he brought them out of their distress.
He stilled the storm to a whisper; the waves of the
sea were hushed.
They were glad when it grew calm, and he guided
them to their desired haven.
Let them give thanks to the Lord for his unfailing
love and his wonderful deeds for mankind.

Gratitude

I am grateful for patient JH and her complete
pathological response, her mother, colleague Christian
Adonizio, a quiet day in the clinic and a quiet post-clinic
treatment room coverage assignment, and home and
rest. I am grateful for a schedule that was not crowded
and for patients who were not ill. I am incredibly
thankful for a house and a family to return to.

Prayer

Lord, I share joy for my patient's complete response. I
pray for comfort for my colleague who is in ill health,
and I pray for an end to suffering for all who are ill.
Grant me insight into breast cancer so that we may
end the scourge if it is your will. Amen.

Today, I believe that the answer is at hand.

What I was doing on this day

There were no medical oncology consultations today. Patient
JH and her mother came to the clinic. She has a *BRCA1*
mutation and triple negative breast cancer. My late doctor

assignment finished at 5:25 PM. I watched movies on my iPad in my office while covering the late clinic. I fell asleep by 9:30 PM at home in front of the television.

Day 35 John 17: 22-23.

I have given them the glory that you gave me, that they may be one as we are one — I in them and you in me — so that they may be brought to complete unity. Then the world will know that you sent me and have loved them even as you have loved me.

Gratitude

I had a marvelous birthday party with Sally, Chris, and our grandchildren. We had rib eye and hamburgers on the grill. The weather was sunny in the 50s. The kids played in the yard. Sally gave me a Garmin D2 Air pilot's watch and a kneeling pad to place on the ground when I sump the fuel tanks in the Cirrus. My sister Louise gave me a Button Up America jigsaw puzzle, filled with presidential campaign buttons from years past. I am grateful for beautiful weather and things that work.

Prayer

Lord, I give you thanks for my manifold blessings. Please grant Heather and Christiaan uncomplicated, peaceful, and prosperous moves. Give our friend Dean clarity of thought; the same goes for pilot Earl. Keep those who fly safe and in your loving care.

Today, I will thank the Lord, for he is good.

What I was doing on this day

I went to Penn Valley Airport to train flight instructors using the Redbird FMX. Dave Hall and Mike Keller were in the FMX for 90 minutes. A physician colleague taking flying lessons was also introduced to the FMX. I reloaded N625VS with its routine contents after its annual inspection. I filled the TKS reservoir with anti-icing fluid. I checked that the transponder was available after the error message, and it worked. I played two *Cargo to Fargo* games with Christiaan and our grandchildren, Lainey, Kade, and Viviaan.

Day 36, my birthday, Psalm 95: 1

> Come, let us sing for joy to the Lord; let us shout aloud to the Rock of our salvation.

Gratitude

> For my 69th birthday, I am in good health with a loving wife and seven grandchildren. I am thankful for a profession and a vocation, a beautiful home, a loving church, and a pleasant community in which we live. I am thankful for friends, family, wealth, and hope. I am thankful for faith in God and in our future. I have much to be thankful for: my health, our family, my wife and children, our grandchildren, and the Engaging Scripture class.

Prayer

> God bless my brother, his wife, and my sister. Grant them continued good health.

Today, I will rejoice in the celebration of another year, a gift from the Lord.

What I was doing on this day

Our son Chris and his kids left at 10 AM. I was too tired to go to church with Sally. She brought home soup made by Chris Zelman. I had a restful day reading and watching TV, The Players Championship at TPC Sawgrass. I reattached the flight deck computer after repairs, and everything worked! I flew multiple instrument approaches at Wildwood Cape May County, Millville, and Atlantic City. I watched *60 Minutes* and *Body of Proof* with Sally. Heather and Stephen called. I spoke to Stephen to invite him to speak at the AOPA STEM teachers' symposium in Orlando in November.

Day 37, Hebrews 4: 12-13

For the word of God is alive and active. Sharper than any double-edged sword, it penetrates even to dividing soul and spirit, joints, and marrow; it judges the thoughts and attitudes of the heart. Nothing in all creation is hidden from God's sight. Everything is uncovered and laid bare before the eyes of him to whom we must give account.

Gratitude

We had a short NAFI board of directors meeting via Zoom. They all wished me a happy birthday, and Bob Meder apologized for not responding to my email saying that I would be at Sun-N-Fun.

Prayer

Thank you, Lord, for granting me clarity of mind as I created my Dropbox video for the upcoming breast cancer webinar.

Today, I will rejoice in the availability of effective cancer treatment for many patients.

What I was doing on this day

It was a busy day in the clinic with a first-year fellow. We had an interesting interaction with a patient who got cervical lymph node swelling after her COVID-19 immunization. There was an even more interesting interaction with her primary care physician about whether the patient needed CT scans and a biopsy. I assured him that she did not because the swelling was due to her COVID-19 vaccination and not to her breast cancer. We had connection problems for our National Accreditation Program of Breast Centers (NAPBC) meeting.

Day 38, Isaiah 40: 11

> He tends his flock like a shepherd: he gathers the lambs in his arms and carries them close to his heart; he gently leads those that have young.

Gratitude

> For a short clinic with few sick patients and a great shrimp curry dinner. Bruce Witkop emailed me to thank me for promoting STEM education in the Central Susquehanna Valley. For Reverend Ryan Krause.

Prayer

> Lord, heal our community, our church, and our nation. Comfort those who fear illness and death and show them the assurances of your care after death.

Today, I will forgive those who offended me.

What I was doing on this day

We had a long discussion at our monthly Presbyterian church Session meeting about opening the library. Should we sing and speak in the sanctuary? Can we have an Easter sunrise service in Veterans Memorial Park? We are awaiting guidance from the borough of Lewisburg. I advocated opening up the building and our worship. Bring back the hymnals (the COVID-19 virus is not spread on fomites), singing, and corporate confession. It was a quiet and reasoned discussion.

Day 39, Colossians 3: 12-15

Therefore, as God's chosen people, holy and dearly loved, clothe yourselves with compassion, kindness, humility, gentleness, and patience. Bear with each other and forgive one another if any of you has a grievance against someone. Forgive as the Lord forgave you. And over all these virtues put on love, which binds them all together in perfect unity.

Let the peace of Christ rule in your hearts since, as members of one body, you were called to peace. And be thankful.

Gratitude

For education and knowledge and opportunity and experience. For peace and few responsibilities. I need a vacation, and one is coming next month when I fly to Florida.

Prayer

Father, grant me an open mind and a clear voice. Cause me to be a voice of love and protection. Guide my words and open the minds and hearts of my listeners. In Jesus' name, Amen.

Today, I will let go, let God.

What I was doing on this day

I gave a talk on breast cancer chemoprevention to a breast cancer webinar based in London. I am enjoying two days off from work to continue my medical education. I spent a very restful day in the Flight Deck reading, filing lessons, and flying approaches on the simulator. Sally made corned beef and cabbage for Saint Patrick's Day. I watched a very well-done documentary about pilot Royal Stratton from Ellwood City, Pennsylvania, who flew a PBY in May 1945 to rescue a B-29 crew downed in Japanese waters.

Day 40, Psalm 90: 12

> Teach us to number our days, that we may gain a heart of wisdom.

Gratitude

> I am grateful for life and learning, knowledge and opportunity, friends and family, Chris and Jessica's buying of a new house, and Heather's ease with her imminent move.

Prayer

> Please help me not to judge those who speak English as their second language. Make me patient with them and cause me to welcome them as strangers, as the Lord directs me to do. Help me to acknowledge their intellect and courage. Please help me to allay their fears.

Today, I will not get angry or wonder why my iPad will neither synchronize nor update.

What I was doing on this day

It is Day 2 of the breast cancer webinar via a Zoom meeting. Understanding many international speakers for whom English is not their first language is challenging. The seminar ended early. I read more than 12 journals and summary pamphlets from the San Antonio breast cancer symposium to catch up on the latest developments in that disease. I reviewed an online meta-analysis of SERM therapy in women with osteopenia or osteoporosis. I watched NCAA basketball with Sally, and Mt. Saint Mary's lost to Texas Southern. Wichita State also lost to Drake. Then, we watched *The Affair*. I am starting to feel sorry for both Allison and Helen.

I am sorry that I am doing too much. I missed Bible study this morning because I was too tired to go and was listening to the continuing medical education seminar.

Day 41, Romans 13: 8

> Let no debt remain outstanding except the continuing debt to love one another, for whoever loves others has fulfilled the law.

Gratitude

> For the relaxation of two days off. For the opportunity to see and to learn, to read and reflect. To write, compose, and create nearly endless opportunities and boundless grace.

Prayer

> Lord, help me love the unlovable: the foolish, selfish, and unwise. To love and forgive those whose love of self is more significant than their love for others. Help me to love the unattractive and the fearful, those who

make excessive demands.

Today, I will strive to understand and love the unloved and to be the Christ they see in the world.

What I was doing on this day

I saw primary care-type patients in the clinic, and I feel it abuses my professional time. An article in the New York *Times* reported large lymph nodes appearing in patients after receiving the COVID-19 vaccine. I showed our secretary, Sadie Stinson, an article in AOPA *Pilot* magazine about a restored 1938 Stinson airplane, a real beauty.

On the consult service, we saw a man with a GIST (gastrointestinal stromal tumor) whose wife wanted a second opinion. A 94-year-old with dementia and colon cancer had a surgical wound abscess. A young African American man with AIDS had Kaposi's sarcoma.

I took my non-working iPad to Best Buy without an appointment, and a member of the Geek Squad said, "We see this all the time. It's so common that Apple pays us to fix them, and we don't charge the customers!" I am astonished.

Day 42, Proverbs 3: 34

He mocks proud mockers but shows favor to the humble and oppressed.

Gratitude

Happy birthday to my sister, Louie! 70! I am glad that the pain in my back and legs was no worse, but I was hobbled. I spoke with Chris; Jessica is pregnant with placenta accreta. Thankfully, her bleeding has stopped.

Prayer

Thank you for solitude and reflection, for the opportunity for quiet thinking, for order in the chaos.

Today, I will try to find time to do nothing.

What I was doing on this day

This evening, three members of Young Life, who were selling mulch as a fundraiser, visited our front door. I invited them in to sit down and told them that I knew Matt Rischel. One of the young women had graduated from Susquehanna University, where Matt went. I told them about Susquehanna STEM to the Skies and gave them my business card and mobile number. I also gave them a check for $100. I flew 90 minutes on the Fly Elite simulator in the Flight Deck.

Day 43, James 1:2-4

Consider it pure joy, my brothers and sisters, whenever you face trials of many kinds, because you know that the testing of your faith produces perseverance. Let perseverance finish its work so that you may be mature and complete, not lacking anything.

Gratitude

I am thankful for Sally and my Cirrus aircraft, my home, and my family. Kathy Storm thanked me for urging the Session to resume singing and speaking during Sunday worship. Sally asked several children to help with the flower boxes at the front of the church.

Prayer

Lord, help me combat evil and know that, with your

help and with prayer, evil can be overcome. Only you can defeat it, but we can send it away. Help me overcome the evil that is breast cancer. In Jesus' name, Amen.

Today, I will thank God for the beautiful weather and a wife who loves me.

What I was doing on this day

I am teaching the Engaging Scripture class today. We are studying Psalm 51 and John 12 ("...the seed must die in the ground and be raised to new life.") I flew the Cirrus in beautiful weather to Reedsville, University Park, Philipsburg, DuBois, and home for a total of 2.4 hours. I did instrument approaches at all the airports except Penn Valley. Sally and I watch the West Virginia University Mountaineers lose a close March Madness game to Syracuse University. I had a deep heart-to-heart talk with Sally. In our talk, we aired old grievances.

Day 44, Psalm 30: 2

Lord my God, I called to you for help, and you healed me.

Gratitude

Jessica is pregnant and has a placenta accreta attached to her cesarean section scar in her uterus. She is bleeding, and her hemoglobin has decreased to 7 grams. She was admitted to Jefferson Hospital and will have a D&C at 9:30 this morning. She is fine. Chris is doing admirably well. For health and wealth, for friends and family. For home and office. For Sally. For the healing of Jessica and the maturity of our son Christiaan.

Prayer

Lord, heal all those who suffer, giving them strength and courage in their hour of need. Make us recall the suffering of Christ on our behalf. Please open my eyes to see the truth of your salvation. In his name. Amen.

Today, I will trust in the healing power of God.

What I was doing on this day

It was a quiet clinic today with our fellow Yvonne Dansoa. We had only one new patient, a Jamaican woman with triple-negative breast cancer. Her daughter, who lives in Harrisburg, was with her and will drive her mother to her clinic appointments. There were no new consultations in the hospital. Sally and I watched Keanu Reeves' movie *A Walk in the Clouds*.

Day 45, Romans 8: 38-39

For I am convinced that neither death nor life, neither angels nor demons, neither the present nor the future, nor any powers, neither height nor depth, nor anything else in all creation, will be able to separate us from the love of God that is in Christ Jesus our Lord.

Gratitude

For a quiet clinic. For a calm colleague (Foghorn). For Sally's care for our family. For Heather and Stephen and the twins. For Jenny Reinhard and Maggie Henderson. For Charity Miller and Christy Gower. For healing of Jessica and Sally's safe trip to Pittsburgh. In quiet solitude and restful sleep.

Prayer

Please help those trying to move Susquehanna STEM to the Skies forward to success.

Today, I will be more diligent in remembering patients' names.

What I was doing on this day

Sally drives to Pittsburgh to be with Chris, Jessica, and the children. Jessica is home, up and about showering. I spent a quiet evening at home. I watched Season One, Episode 5 of *Luther*, in which John and Alice resolve Ian's murder of Chloe. I fell asleep watching a movie. During the clinic day, I worked on a PowerPoint presentation about thunderstorms.

Day 46, 2 Samuel 22: 33-34

It is God who arms me with strength and keeps my way secure. He makes my feet like the feet of a deer; He causes me to stand on the heights.

Gratitude

Sally tells me about Ladies in Flight Training, www. flylift.org. I share this with one of my female flight students. I am thankful for the time available to run errands.

Prayer

Bring healing to Jessica and a rapid sale of their house. Lord, show me how to end breast cancer.

What I was doing on this day

Dan Carlson and I see a woman who has triple negative breast cancer and thyrotoxicosis from one of her cancer treatment drugs. I leave the hospital rounds at 3:00 PM and stop at the grocery store. Then, I stopped at the hardware store to buy bird seed. Then, I went to the Country Cupboard to purchase pies and cakes for the office tomorrow. I am grateful for the opportunity to serve others.

Day 47, John 10: 9-11

I am the gate; whoever enters through me will be saved. They will come in and go out and find pasture. The thief comes only to steal, kill, and destroy; I have come that they may have life and have it to the full. I am the Good Shepherd. The good shepherd lays down his life for the sheep.

Gratitude

A young flight instructor called to inquire about my STEM to the Skies plans. I am thankful for many of my colleagues at work.

Prayer

Soften the heart of a colleague and make him more sensitive and receptive to the opinions of others.

Today, I will thank God for my health.

What I was doing on this day

I lead Bible study on 2 Chronicles 27-31. We celebrated a colleague's birthday at the office. A Taco truck comes to the clinic. A 27-year-old woman started chemotherapy. I fell asleep watching another episode of Luther. Sally called from Pittsburgh to report two showings of Chris and Jessica's house. There is a video of our grandson Maverick at the dentist. I am praying for the healing of several friends. I am grateful for the nurses in my clinic and for Sally.

Day 48, Psalm 12: 7

You, Lord, will keep the needy safe and protect us forever from the wicked.

Gratitude

One of our young physician assistants is becoming knowledgeable and competent in medical oncology. This evening, there is a beautiful moonrise.

Prayer

Thank you, Lord, for my manifold blessings: wife, children, grandchildren. For my career, for aviation, for aviation podcasts, for aviation publications and their editors.

What I was doing on this day

Today, I will rejoice at my many gifts and abilities and the opportunity to serve others. The late doctor ends at 5:30 PM. I smoked a cigar on the front porch. I listened to Billy Joel and Bonnie Raitt on Sirius XM radio. One of our patients had severe neutropenia and diarrhea, along with pharyngitis and dehydration. There are only two new consultations. One was a man with non-small cell lung cancer. Another patient has oral cancer.

Day 49, 1 Peter 3: 15-16

But in your hearts, revere Christ as Lord. Always be prepared to answer everyone who asks you and give the reason for your hope. But do this with gentleness and respect, keeping a clear conscience, so that those who speak maliciously against your good behavior in Christ may be ashamed of their slander.

Gratitude

I am grateful for the Cirrus, the excellent weather, and for spending the day with family and returning home. I watched the German movie drama *The Captain*. It is a superb historical, moral tale.

Prayer

For food, for raiment,
For life, for opportunity,
For friendship and fellowship,
We thank thee, O Lord. Amen

Today, I will rejoice in my grandchildren.

What I was doing on this day

Sally has spent the week in Canonsburg with Chris, Jessica, and the grandchildren. They have sold their house. I flew to the Washington County airport in glorious weather and joined them all at the Print Scape ice arena at South Point to watch Kade's hockey practice. We had lunch at Bubba's Burgers. We returned to the house with Sally and Finnegan while all the others got haircuts. Due to opposing traffic, I flew back at 11,000 feet per air traffic control request. My Garmin D2 Air watch said my oxygen saturation was 94%. There was a curious carbon monoxide alarm three times from my Sentry receiver. I felt fine. My O2 saturation was greater than 92%. I suspect it was a false alarm. I am eager to teach others to fly.

Day 50, Palm Sunday, Deuteronomy 4: 7

What other nation is so great as to have their gods near them the way the Lord our God is near us whenever we pray to him?

Gratitude

Reverend Ryan Krause preached an exceptional Palm Sunday sermon on Psalm 118 and Mark 11. It was a quiet Palm Sunday, and the sermon was excellent, Reverend Krause noting that the Palm Sunday celebration was premature.

Prayer

May our loud hosannas never forget the pain of the cross. Today, I will enjoy the time off.

What was I doing this day?

Sally returned home. I started the day at the Engaging Scripture Zoom class, then watched the church service on YouTube. I made a list of all the airports listed in my first logbook.

Day 51, Hebrews 10: 22

Let us draw near to God with a sincere heart and with the full assurance that faith brings, having our hearts sprinkled to cleanse us from a guilty conscience and having our bodies washed with pure water.

Gratitude

For a loving wife. For a pleasant defense attorney from Indianapolis whom I spoke with about a case of delayed diagnosis of breast cancer.

Prayer

For two physicians who are defendants in a malpractice suit and for the patient's family in question.

Today, I will rejoice that my colleague has returned to do hospital consultations.

What I was doing on this day?

My fellow is not in the clinic because she has to attend a vital meeting. Another fellow said the meeting was about delivering bad news to patients and families. It lasted four hours and was conducted with actors who were playing patients. One of our fellows joined me in the Breast Multidisciplinary Clinic. A brilliant medical student from the Philadelphia College of Osteopathic Medicine joined us. She answered all my questions about clinical epidemiology.

Day 51, Psalm 121: 1-2

I left up my eyes to the hills—where does my help come from? My help comes from the Lord, the maker of heaven and earth.

Gratitude

I need to organize my desk at home early in the morning. I have only five patients and a 3:00 PM departure from the office, so I need to start at 8:30 a.m. in the clinic.

Prayer

Thank you, Lord, for healthy patients today and the opportunity to get to the airport for 90 minutes.

Today, I will be more grateful and optimistic.

I left the office before 3:00 and bought 13 bagels at Panera Bread in the Tuesday half-price sale. I then went to the airport to leave a key for the simulator for one of the flight instructors. I met Dr. Tom Bowen and Dirk Lander, who owns a Cessna 210. I showed them the Redbird FMX simulator. Flight instructor Dave Hall had just finished with a student in the simulator. I also met a young man who owns a Mooney airplane and works with his father in a family concrete finishing business.

Day 52, Galatians 4: 7

So, you are no longer a slave but God's child, and since you are his child, God has also made you an heir.

Gratitude

For a vice president at the bank who set up credit card billing for my STEM program.

Prayer

I'm grateful for friends who worship with us at church, for friends who own a bed and breakfast in our town, for our children, Heather and Christiaan, for Stephen and Jessica and "the seven," for work colleagues, and for our pastor, Reverend Ryan Krause.

Today, I will look for opportunities to serve.

What the Geisinger Health System needs to provide:

1. Respect for its physicians.
2. To put physicians in charge of program
3. To develop centers of excellence
4. To promote and require close collaborations and team building among disparate medical disciplines
5. To pair physicians with mid-level practitioners in

      ongoing one-on-one relationships

6. To create follow-up clinics organized by disease sites
7. To place doctoral-level clinical psychologists in the clinics every day
8. To bring continuing medical education back onto the campus and not just via the Internet
9. To develop positive, rather than negative, physician incentives
10. To analyze and publish disease outcomes for individual physicians in physician subspecialty groups.

I had a long discussion today along with one of our fellows and our lead physician assistant with a 61-year-old woman with a 10-centimeter small cell lung cancer.

Day 53, Maundy Thursday, Ephesians 4: 29

Do not let any unwholesome talk come out of your mouths, but only what helps build others up according to their needs so that they may benefit those who listen.

Gratitude

Happy birthday, Uncle Don! I left the clinic at 11:00 AM and drove to the airport. I met M&T Bank vice president Heather Buttorff and gave her a demonstration ride in the Redbird FMX simulator. The bank needed to verify that we are a public charity and that we really own the simulator.

Prayer

Lord, grant success to our STEM effort. Open the hearts and minds of all local school administrators and teachers to our program and the opportunities it presents. Bless Glenn Ponas and Karla Smith in their outreach efforts from the Aircraft Owners and Pilots Association.

Today, I will embrace the burden of washing the feet of others.

Our son Chris moved his bed and other household belongings in a rented U-Haul to their new house in Elizabethtown today. He came to our house late last night with Lainey, Kade, and Viviaan (three of his five children). Sally and I watched the Maundy Thursday church service on YouTube. Chris and three of his children drove to Cannonsburg for a friend of Lainey's birthday party. Jessica took Sally's car to work in York.

Pastor Krause's Maundy Thursday sermon focused on washing feet more than on the darkness of Gethsemane.

Day 54, Good Friday, II Corinthians 5:8

I say we are confident and would prefer to be away from the body and at home with the Lord.

Gratitude

I remember fondly eating Easter candy from the Wolfgang Candy company in York, Pennsylvania, as a child. I also remember Easter dinner with my grandparents, my boyhood friend Delbert, and the neighborhood pond, where we spent many hours. I recall fondly Good Friday services as a child that lasted from noon to 3:00 PM, with seven pastors each conducting a 30-minute service on the seven last words of Christ from the cross.

Prayer

> May we never forget the price paid for our forgiveness and salvation because God loves us. I am thankful to be mindful of propitiation and the expiation of my sins.

Today, I will thank God for forgiveness in his manifold blessings that he showers upon me.

Sally took me to work with Kade and Viviaan because Jessica has her car. Chris arrived in Lewisburg with his other three children. In the morning, I saw treatment patients in the clinic and talked with an attorney for whom I provided expert testimony in a malpractice case. We did three hospital consultations, and Sally picked me up by 3:30. We had dinner with Chris and his children. I was in bed by 9:30.

Day 55, Psalm 103: 2-5

> Praise the Lord, my soul, and
> forget not all his benefits—
> who forgives all your sins
> and heals all your diseases,
> who redeems your life from the pit
> and crowns you with love and
> compassion,
> who satisfies your desires with
> good things
> so that your youth is renewed like
> the eagle's.

Gratitude

> We give you thanks for laughing children and a loving son, for son-in-law and daughter-in-law who love us, and for our children and their children, our

grandchildren. We give you thanks for rest, peace, and hope.

Prayer

Lord, may we always remember those darkest days when all hope seemed lost, promises were broken, and hopes were shattered. Let us never forget what followed the crucifixion, and may we always trust in the hope and power of the resurrection.

Today, I will remember both the promise and the reality of the resurrection.

This is the darkest day of the year. He was filled with such hope and promise. He performed miracles and told the good news. We all believed in him. Then, those who could not match his deeds of loving kindness killed him because they saw him as a threat to their power and control. Those who were incompetent plotted against and killed the most competent man who ever lived. Envy, vainglory, and hypocrisy killed this kind, loving teacher who showed us all a better way. But now, the world was even darker than before; our hopes were dashed, and our lives were in danger. Why has God forsaken us?

One of our granddaughters thought the Easter story was "funny" when her mother explained it to her. Perhaps even children can no longer come to Jesus.

Day 56, Easter Sunday, Matthew 28: 5-7.

The angel said to the women, "Do not be afraid, for I know you are looking for Jesus, who was crucified. He is not here; he has risen, just as he said. Come and see the place where he lay. Then go quickly and tell his disciples: 'He has risen from the dead and is going ahead of you into Galilee. There you will see him.' Now I have told you."

Gratitude

For the greatest gift of all, the Resurrection. Hallelujah! For health and family, work and recreation, and the promise of eternal life.

Prayer

Lord, thank you for the resurrection. While we were sinners, you loved us and gave us eternal life as a gift we did not earn.

Today, I will Trust in the Lord and hope for the future.

Christiaan and the kids are here. We had sunrise service in Soldiers and Sailors Park and good attendance. Two high school students played hymns, one with the trumpet and the other with the saxophone. We went to church and sang. COVID-19 has passed. What an incredible difference from last year! We had Easter dinner with Christiaan and the children. It was a beautiful day outside with children, an egg hunt, and a kite. I built a pink cottage for Viviaan and played Cargo to Fargo with Chris, Lainey, and Kade. God is present in our families.

Day 57, Easter Monday, Proverbs 13: 20

Walk with the wise and become wise, for a companion of fools suffers harm.

Gratitude

For the grace of the Resurrection and the joy of family. I am now enjoying the peace of a home without five grandchildren.

Prayer

Slow me down, Lord, let me know that this is your world.

Today, I will rejoice in a family-filled Easter weekend.

Jessica returned Sally's car this morning after working in York since Thursday. She, Christiaan, and the children returned to Pittsburgh this morning.

Day 58, 1 John 5:18

We know that anyone born of God does not continue to sin; the one born of God keeps them safe, and the evil one cannot harm them.

Gratitude

I had a gentle schedule today at my Lewisburg clinic but had little time to write this week.

Prayer

Lord, help me to be less anxious about all the details in preparing for next week and our trip to Florida. May I trust in your sheltering hand.

Today, I will Rejoice in God's grace.

Susquehanna STEM to the Skies board of directors meeting today. Three of our board members are away with illness or travel. I am concerned that the STEM program is not moving forward more quickly. I need to create a more structured development plan for the STEM program.

Day 59, Psalm 36: 7

How priceless is your unfailing love, O God! People take refuge in the shadow of your wings.

Gratitude

For Seth and Judith Ziegler, for Doug and Cindy Fischer. For only one hospital consult today.

Prayer

Please provide health and recovery to my patient and guidance with success for her son, who is pursuing an aviation career.

Today, I will rejoice at opportunities.

I met a nurse from our hospital who will now be my patient. She has locally advanced breast cancer. I am concerned about her prognosis. We had only one hospital consult: a young man with the human immunodeficiency virus (HIV) who has cancer and declined chemotherapy. He received radiation only, and now he has progressive disease. We had dinner with Cindy and Doug Fischer at Ziegler's house. A very pleasant evening.

Day 60, Revelation 1: 5-6

… and from Jesus Christ, who is the faithful witness, the firstborn from the dead, and the ruler of the kings of the earth. To him who loves us and has freed us from our sins by his blood and has made us a kingdom and priests to serve his God and Father—to him be glory and power forever and ever! Amen.

Gratitude

I am grateful for the opportunity to create the Susquehanna Valley STEM program and to serve NAFI on its board of directors and at the Sun-N-Fun fly-in in Lakeland, FL.

Prayer

Bring peace to my colleague and his wife, who has atrial fibrillation. Help the colleague who suffers from obsessive-compulsive disorder and grant her peace and solace in the coming days.

Today, I will rejoice in fond memories of playing golf with friends.

I met a couple who live in Montoursville. He was a professional golfer, and she had a good prognosis for her breast cancer. One of our nurses tells me that her son is a high school junior interested in an aviation career. Glenn Ponas from AOPA spoke with Colleen Epler-Ruths at the CSIU, along with her supervisor, about our STEM program. CSIU is curious but does not know how to operationalize a STEM program. We had a training webinar for NAFI regarding the upcoming annual fly-in at Lakeland called Sun-N-Fun.

Day 61, Proverbs 14: 29

Whoever is patient has great understanding, but one who is quick-tempered displays folly.

Gratitude

For a late morning clinic schedule and for two nurses, Jennie and Joann, who educate and comfort my patients.

Prayer

Lord, guide my thoughts and words so that I may bring others to love and serve you. May others see your grace in me.

Today, I believe that God will reveal the mystery of breast cancer to me in his time.

I spent the early morning cleaning my desk of STEM issues and receipts for taxes, and I printed and copied essential documents. I finished clinic patients by 11:30. I spent 45 minutes during my NCI- RCR (Registration and Credential Repository) renewal. We saw three very sick patients: my patient with extensive lung, liver, and bone metastases; a patient of a colleague of mine with small cell lung cancer and multiple brain metastases; and a patient from another institution in Williamsport with lung metastases who was breathing with high- flow nasal oxygen. The Lord was with me, our physician assistant, and our first-year fellow as we delivered sad news to our dying patients.

Day 62, Romans 8: 37

No, in all these things we are more than conquerors through him who loved us.

Gratitude

For the Redbird FMX simulator and the STEM to the Skies program. I received a surprise e-mail from dentist Dr. Carl Jenkins, a pilot who thoroughly enjoyed his time in our simulator. I am treating breast cancer in one of his dental hygienists.

Prayer

> Lord, help me believe that the STEM program will succeed. Open the minds and hearts of teachers and administrators to its possibilities.

Today, I trust that others will come to recognize the value of STEM education in our area.

Our Engaging Scripture class studied John 20 and 1, 2 John. Sally and I watched an exciting day three at the Masters golf tournament, with Hideki Matsuyama being the first Japanese golfer to lead the tournament. He would thus be the first to win. Then, Sally and I watched *News of the World* with Tom Hanks and young Helena Zengel.

Day 63, Psalm 29: 11

> The Lord gives strength to his people, and the Lord blesses his people with peace.

Gratitude

> For Ryan Krause, our Engaging Scripture class, Amber Lind and David Shrom, and Sally and her unassuming love of others. We enjoyed Ryan Krause's sermons on John 20 and 1 John 3.

Prayer

> Lord, give us safe passage to Florida. Bless Stephen and Heather in their move and Christiaan and Jessica in theirs.

Today, I will fear no evil.

I am reading *The Undercover God*, a book about modern Gnostics. I enjoyed a relaxing day at home. Sally delivered flowers for the Presbyterian deacons. I cleared four months of reading material in the Flight Deck and watched the *Band of Brothers* episode in which they liberated a concentration camp.

Day 64, Matthew 11: 28-30

Come to me, all you who are weary and burdened, and I will give you rest. Take my yoke upon you and learn from me, for I am gentle and humble in heart, and you will find rest for your souls. For my yoke is easy and my burden is light.

Gratitude

For flyable weather from Selinsgrove through northern Virginia. For a beautiful evening flight from Columbia, SC, to the Jacksonville Executive Airport. For Stephen coming to pick us up at the airport. We are grateful for helping hands at the airports where we land.

Prayer

Thank you, Lord, for safety as we fly.

Today, I will trust in the Lord.

I finished the clinic on time. I left the Breast Multidisciplinary Clinic early. We got to Penn Valley Airport before 3:00 PM and departed at 3:30. We had a bumpy ride through Virginia and North Carolina to Columbia, South Carolina.

Day 65, Isaiah 44: 22

I have swept away your offenses like a cloud, your sins like the morning mist. Return to me, for I have redeemed you.

Gratitude

For travel that develops and unfolds as planned. For a quiet, peaceful morning in Heather and Stephen's lanai.

Prayer

Thank you, Lord, for sheltering me under your protective wings.

Today, I will be grateful for flying, family and friends, health and safety.

I flew to Bartow, Florida, in clear but turbulent weather. As I flew from Jacksonville to Bartow, the clouds were swept away. I met the same couple from Michigan as I had met two years ago. I drove the rental car to the home of Dr. Leonard Gitter, a beautiful house. I met his mother and father, who are from Ukraine. Leo took me out to dinner, and we talked for hours.

Day 66, Luke 17: 3-4

So, watch yourselves. "If your brother or sister sins against you, rebuke them; and if they repent, forgive them. Even if they sin against you seven times in a day and seven times come back to you saying, 'I repent,' you must forgive them."

Gratitude

It was a fabulous day at Sun-N-Fun, filled with discussions about STEM. I did not get sunburned! I walked and walked and didn't overeat.

Prayer

Lord, look with mercy and grace on Matthew Lynch, Brian Hughes, Jamie Becket, Mike Zidziunas, Mission Aviation Fellowship, JAARS, and all aviation training programs. Open their students to the opportunities available to them.

Today, I will be grateful for opportunities.

I listened to an excellent lecture at noon by Jamie Beckett from AOPA, who talked about flying clubs. I spoke with him for 20 minutes after his presentation. I met Brian Hughes from Winter Haven, who founded the *Aspiring Aviator's Aero-Club*. I then talked to Mike Zidziunas at the Lakeland Aero Club and saw their FMX simulator. I gathered great gifts for our grandchildren. There was a delightful session at JD Deboskey's T-34, where John and Martha King joined us for pictures. I took long walks on the grounds. I visited Jungle Aviation and Relay Service (JAARS) and Mission Aviation Fellowship and flew a Quest Kodiak virtual simulator. I met Rachel and her children from JAARS at JD Deboskey's T-34 airplane.

Day 67, Psalm 146: 7

He upholds the cause of the oppressed and gives food to the hungry. The Lord sets prisoners free.

Gratitude

For good weather and good lectures. For Bob Meder and NAFI. For friendship and responsibility in bringing about the next generation of pilots.

Prayer

Lord, guard and guide the men and women who fly.

Today, I will rejoice at the gift of medical radiation.

I attended three excellent lectures in the morning. Rachel Stoner spoke about JAARS and the Mission Aviation Fellowship founders. Gary Reeves talked about using autopilots in IFR flights, and Martin Pauly explained in detail how he produces GoPro videos in his Bonanza. The afternoon air show was excellent. I spent time with Bob Meder at the NAFI booth. I enjoyed a pizza dinner with Leo Gitter.

Day 68, 1 Corinthians 6: 19

Do you not know that your bodies are temples of the Holy Spirit, who is in you, whom you have received from God? You are not your own.

Gratitude

I had cheese Danish for breakfast at Sun-N-Fun and a fried lobster roll for lunch. I attended an excellent lecture on flying to Canada and spoke with Richard McSpadden after his excellent talk on risk management.

Prayer

Lord, bring peace and comfort to the Gitter home. Bring resolution to Leo and his wife. Grant Adam your tender care.

Today, I will rejoice in my many gifts from God.

I attended a press conference with the NAFI and King Schools along with the first scholarship winner and Robert Meder, immediate past president of NAFI. I told the audience that you really don't know something until you can teach it. I spent the afternoon at the NAFI booth, where we had good interest from flight instructors. Unfortunately, the Internet was not working well. I had dinner alone at the Outback Steakhouse and was in bed by 9:20. Leo and his parents were meeting Adam at the airport.

Day 69, Proverbs 12: 17

An honest witness tells the truth, but a false witness tells lies.

Gratitude

I spent the morning with Dave Conner, a flight instructor from the Bronx at the NAFI booth. There were overcast skies with rain showers but no thunderstorms. I left the NAFI booth and flew pleasantly from Bartow Airport to the Jacksonville Executive Airport. Sally, Heather, and the twins picked me up. We had a delicious salmon dinner with Heather and Steve.

Prayer

Lord, bless Heather and Steve in this time of transition. If it is your will, bring new opportunities to Dave Conner.

Today, I will play with my grandchildren.

I had a long conversation with Dave Conner, who was 35 when he got his high school graduate equivalent degree. He was working as a truck driver and then began to fly. He teaches at the Orlando Executive Airport and wants to enter corporate aviation. Tom Huitema and his girlfriend Desiree stop by the NAFI booth. He flies a Boeing 787 for American Airlines. There was a huge crowd this Saturday at Sun-N-Fun despite the pandemic. I am grateful that all my travel has gone smoothly.

Day 70, Luke 12: 32

Do not be afraid, little flock, for your father has been pleased to give you the Kingdom.

Gratitude

The ceiling at the Jacksonville Executive Airport was 800 feet overcast, but the winds were light, and the thunderstorms were well off to the South. Loading the Cirrus in light rain was easy, and the departure was not delayed. There was significant mist on the windscreen, which cleared quickly with the defroster. We had no turbulence on the flight to the Southern Pines Airport in North Carolina.

Prayer

We thank you for safe travel and cooperative weather, Oh Lord. Thank you for the privilege of flying and safety on our travels.

Today, I will delight in our freedom to fly.

We left the Jacksonville Executive Airport on the northern edge of a west-to-east drooping warm front, with light rain and 800-foot overcast skies to the north. There were thunderstorms to the south over Ormond Beach. The ride between Brunswick and Savannah was smooth for us in clear air. We stopped at the Southern Pines airport and paid $5.99 per gallon for fuel, then picked up Dr. Russell Stankiewicz at Lancaster Airport in Pennsylvania. He was dropping off his Cirrus for its annual inspection. The total flight time for the trip to Sun-N-Fun in Lakeland, Florida, was 12.1 hours.

Day 71, Psalm 42: 5-6

Why, my soul, are you downcast? Why so disturbed within me? Put your hope in God, for I will yet praise him, my Savior and my God. My soul is downcast within me; Therefore, I will remember you from the land of Jordan, the heights of Hermon from Mount Mizar.

Gratitude

I am grateful for the job I am returning to and for the colleagues who watched over my patients in my absence last week. I quickly cleared 158 items in my inbox, and for easy patients in the Breast Cancer Multidisciplinary Clinic.

Prayer

For all those who serve the sick, give them tenderness and insight, Oh Lord. Bring your healing and nurturing power to their hands. May others see your grace in them. In the name of the great physician, Amen.

Today, I will rejoice in the opportunity to bring hope and healing through God's grace.

There are only two new patients in the multidisciplinary clinic, but there were very ill patients on consult rounds, including a very jaundiced 95-year-old man with a serum bilirubin of 21. He had cancer of the pancreas. I am exhausted at home after the week in Florida.

Day 72, Revelation 22: 5

There will be no more night. They will not need the light of a lamp or the light of the sun, for the Lord God will give them light. And they will reign forever and ever.

Gratitude

I am amazed each day that there is so much to be thankful for and for this opportunity to record my thoughts. I received a very encouraging e-mail from Glenn Ponas at AOPA about his progress with the CSIU.

Prayer

Lord, help me acknowledge my weaknesses and seek your help daily. Lead me to your truth and grant me the blessings of knowledge and insight, if it be your will, so that I will bring healing to your people.

Today, I will rejoice in many demands and opportunities.

Two patients for whom I've cared for a very long time are experiencing progressive disease. Wanda has muscle weakness and fatigue from her whole brain radiation therapy and her oral steroids. Wilimina has progressive lymphedema and skin lesions. I will change her chemotherapy. The Session meeting at church runs long until 9:00 PM. There are many procedural issues. Reverend Barbara Yorks will be the new Himmelreich librarian. The NAFI board meeting is again focused on finances primarily and needs a strategic vision. I believe that one of its employees has adult attention deficit disorder.

Day 73, Isaiah 46: 4

Even to your old age and gray hair, I am he; I am he who will sustain you. I have made you, and I will carry you, sustain you, and rescue you.

Gratitude

Last evening, one of my colleagues advised me that one of our fellows had to be in a meeting and would miss the first 90 minutes of our morning clinic. I saw three not-so-ill patients. I spoke with one of my favorite patients and her husband following her first chemotherapy last week for her newly diagnosed triple-negative breast cancer.

Prayer

Please bring comfort and solace to all those in our care and the women we counseled in the cancer genetics clinic today. Ease their fears and show them your presence. In Jesus' name, Amen.

Today, I will reach out in Christian compassion to my patient's son.

We had a lengthy cancer genetics high-risk clinic today with five patients, one of whom was only 24 years old. The medical oncology fellow and I had a difficult conversation with one of our patients and her sisters regarding her progressive breast cancer.

The NAFI *Mentor Live* session this evening was canceled because our president did not agree with the slides of the presenter, who was an instrument flight instructor and attorney who discussed the ABCs of FAA enforcement actions. The NAFI president did not indicate what he found to be objectionable.

Day 74, Psalm 65: 9

You care for the land and water it; you enrich it

abundantly. The streams of God are filled with water to provide the people with grain, for so you have ordained it.

Gratitude

Eric Schmidt led Bible study for Tom Gresh, Bill Morrow, and me. After today, one of our best outpatient clerical assistants will leave the clinic. It was a blissfully uneventful day, and I enjoyed the peaceful quiet of my office.

Prayer

Lord, heal the wife of my colleague of her heart disease and ease my colleague's troubled mind. Please hasten her recovery so they may visit Florida for rest and recuperation.

Today, I will admit my sin of not loving those who are unattractive and offensive at times.

Day 75, Psalm 30: 6-7

When I felt secure, I said, "I will never be shaken." Lord, when you favored me, you made my royal mountain stand firm, but when you hid your face, I was dismayed.

Gratitude

I am pleased when patients are well. I am delighted with my collaborative nurse and the care she provides for my patients.

Prayer

God, grant relief of suffering to those in physical

pain and comfort to those in spiritual distress. Bless the gay man in the intensive care unit with the new tracheostomy and an upper aerodigestive tumor. Lord, make me love the unattractive sinner.

Today, I will be thankful that I can serve others.

I spoke with a representative of a large international pharmaceutical firm and her medical liaison officer. They have a new drug for metastatic HER2-positive breast cancer. We exchanged anecdotes about a colleague of mine who shares my last name. I was called to the treatment room at 5:15 PM to see the patient of a colleague who has follicular lymphoma. She is being treated with a chemotherapy drug and an immunological agent. She has a fever of 102 degrees Fahrenheit and an absolute neutrophil count of 560. She needs to be admitted to the hospital for antibiotic treatment of neutropenic fever. When I told the patient's husband, "Yes, she will be alright," he had tears in his eyes.

Day 76, Romans 2: 1-3

You, therefore, have no excuse, you who passed judgment on someone else, for at whatever point you judge another, you are condemning yourself because you who passed judgment do the same things. Now we know that God's judgment against those who do such things is based on truth. So, when you, a mere human being, pass judgment on them and yet do the same things, do you think you will escape God's judgment?

Gratitude

I am so thankful to be a flight instructor and to have the opportunity to teach and serve.

Prayer

Thank you for Dr. Carl Jenkins. May his enthusiasm inspire others to value STEM education and open the minds of the WRAP members and the Civil Air Patrol to the value of simulator training.

Today, I will rejoice in the gift of flight.

Today, I flew for an hour in the Redbird FMX simulator with Dr. Carl Jenkins, a local dentist. He was as excited as a child. We flew the ILS to runway 27 at Williamsport and then went to Altus, Oklahoma, where his daughter is an Air Force pilot learning to fly the C-17. He sent a very kind e-mail thank you afterward. His dental assistant is a patient of mine. Then I saw the son of another of my patients, and we flew in the simulator, followed by a flight in my Cirrus. Sally and I watched *It's Complicated*.

Day 77, Proverbs 18: 24

One with unreliable friends comes to ruin, but a friend sticks closer than a brother.

Gratitude

For Tom and Nancy Neilson, who have enjoyed joining our Engaging Scripture class, a quiet and restful day at home and an hour and a half on the Fly Elite simulator.

Prayer

For the health of the church and the vitality of the public health. Remove the fears of illness from the hearts of your people and return us to normal as soon as it is your will. In his name, Amen.

Today, I will enjoy the rest of the Sabbath.

Ryan Krause delivered a thoughtful sermon today, noting that the epistles of John contain more uses of the word "love" than any other gospels or epistles. I wrote to Gus Putsche at NAFI explaining that the CDC has removed surface disinfecting protocols. I asked that we not do that at Air Venture with our Redbird simulators between lessons. I had a delightful broasted chicken dinner at the Country Cupboard Restaurant.

Day 78, Matthew 23: 12

Those who exalt themselves will be humbled, and those who humble themselves will be exalted.

Gratitude

For food, for raiment,
For life, for opportunity,
For friendship and fellowship,
We thank thee, O Lord.

Prayer

Bring healing to all those in my care. Bless our first-year fellow and her coming marriage. Bless Christiaan, Jessica, and the children moving from Pittsburgh to Elizabethtown. Regard Stephen, Heather, and the twins with tender compassion. Vouchsafe to guard them under your wing.

Today, I will Rejoice in God's grace.

My sleep-wake cycle is at its ebb. Sally fixed a leak in the washing machine, and I installed five hooks on a board in my closet. We had leftovers for dinner. A colleague did hospital medical oncology consultations, and I was home by 4:15 PM. I spent a quiet evening in front of the television and was in bed by 10:00 o'clock.

Day 79, Psalm 18: 34-35

He trains my hands for battle; my arms can bend a bow of bronze. You make your saving help my shield, and your right hand sustains me; your help has made me great.

Gratitude

Due to a scheduling glitch, there are only five patients in the clinic today. I spoke with BJ Teichman, the airport manager at Bloomsburg, about promoting STEM education in our region.

Prayer

Today, Lord, make me strong. Make today the day that you revealed to me the mystery that is breast cancer so that I may bring your grace to your people and end their suffering. Thy will be done.

Today, I will use my time wisely to recreate.

Mundane tasks were required today. My SUV got an oil change, new front wiper blades, and a replacement fuel pressure valve. The old valve prevented remote starts with the key fob. My optimism about our STEM program rises and falls, depending on whom I talk to.

Day 80, 2 Peter 1: 3

His divine power has given us everything we need for a godly life through our knowledge of him who called us by his own glory and goodness.

Gratitude

I'm grateful for nurses and secretaries who make me laugh, a physician assistant who has served us well and is now moving on, and a radiologist and mammographer for being friends. I'm also glad for the smiles of our nurses, who were grateful for the ice cream we brought them.

Prayer

Lord, make today the day that you reveal your secrets to me. Please guide me to the knowledge that will end the suffering if it be your will, in Jesus' name. Amen.

Today, I will listen to that still small voice.

Sally and I watched Ken Burns' *Hemingway* series on PBS. Hemingway was a fascinating and highly talented man who, critics, historians, and scholars say, single-handedly changed the face of American literature. He was the greatest American writer since Mark Twain. He was also an adulterer, having four wives, who "fell in love with the next woman before he left the current one."

Day 81, Jeremiah 32: 40

I will make an everlasting covenant with them; I will never stop doing good to them, and I will inspire them to fear me so that they will never turn away from me.

Gratitude

I finished with my last patient at 3:30 PM. A few new patients were in the clinic, and I shared them with our physician assistant. Unfortunately, my Foghorn colleague talked incessantly. I was disappointed that the CSIU would not agree to a visit. I spoke with NAFI president Bob Meder about my role in NAFI and where the organization needs to go. He asked me to speak with one of the board members and one of the NAFI employees for guidance and clarification. I made approaches on the Elite simulator at Appleton, WI, in preparation for our trip to Oshkosh and AirVenture 2021.

Prayer

Please guide me in moving our STEM program forward and grant me patience.

Today, I will rejoice in being the late doctor.

Day 82, II Corinthians 1: 20

No matter what promises God has made, they are "Yes" in Christ. And so through him the "Amen" is spoken by us to the glory of God.

Gratitude

I watched a historical fiction account entitled *Six Minutes to Midnight* about German girls in an English boarding school. They were German spies being groomed by the Nazis. Judy Dench portrayed the headmistress. It is an exciting story. A patient who is diabetic and an amputee chose to stop her chemotherapy after only two of four prescribed cycles were administered. Her disease extended beyond the capsule of her axillary lymph nodes, a very poor prognostic sign. We are condemned by sin and freed by grace.

Prayer

> For the patient with the mesothelioma and his wife who seems not to grasp the contribution of his cigarette smoking to both his cancer and his chronic obstructive pulmonary disease. May he not suffer significantly as he dies, and may he know the Lord.

Today, I will enjoy being the late doctor in the medical oncology clinic.

Day 83, Psalm 33: 4

> For the word of the Lord is right and true; He is faithful in all he does.

Gratitude

> For health and home, for friends and colleagues and daily food, and for the special knowledge that I possess as a flight instructor. The sun was glorious this morning, and I took photographs of our flowering cherry trees in the front yard.

Prayer

> Lord, make me faithful in all that I do. May I seek and acknowledge you so that you may direct my paths. Bring financial security to NAFI and may Oshkosh AirVenture 2021 be a great success.

Today, I will vow to write like Ernest Hemingway. Not to live like him, but to write like him!

My iPhone will not download pictures to my computer, and

I cannot load them to OneDrive or to the cloud. It is very frustrating. I had a restful day at home. Sally and I worked on the campaign button jigsaw puzzle my sister Louise gave us.

Day 84, James 4: 8

Come near to God, and he will come near to you. Wash your hands, you sinners, and purify your hearts, you double-minded.

Gratitude

For a day of rest. For pleasant weather. For our Engaging Scripture class. For sister Louise and brother Tim. It is good to know the Lord.

Prayer

Please keep our family safe in your tender care. Protect us from harm and lead us to seek your will. We thank you for all your blessings. Guide us to help those in need. In Jesus' name, Amen.

Today, I will continue working on "The Exam Room," a play that exposes the folly and suffering of current cancer treatment.

We finished the jigsaw puzzle, took a picture, and sent it to Louise. We spoke to her on the phone for an hour. I met with Josh Maciejewski at Penn Valley Airport and discussed our STEM program for an hour. He and his wife Brianna are on the Southern Columbia school board. He is quite interested in getting a STEM education program at Southern Columbia High School. His company, *Function of Beauty*, is worth millions and is about either to go public or to be sold.

Day 85, Proverbs 13: 11

Dishonest money dwindles away, but whoever gathers money little by little makes it grow.

Gratitude

I'm grateful that I have gathered money little by little and had the opportunity to be generous. Generosity has grown my monetary blessings.

Prayer

Lord, grant healing to those who suffer. Bring relief to them and rest to their souls. Comfort their spouses and children.

Today, I will be thankful for the opportunity to serve others.

Our clinic was packed this morning, and our first-year fellow blessed them and me. We wrestled with confusing questions in the Breast Multidisciplinary Clinic. A young surgeon and her lack of experience presented particular challenges. There was only one hospital consultation to see at 4:15 PM. God showed up today in the exam rooms and the hearts and minds of troubled patients.

Day 86, Revelation 2: 11

Whoever has ears, let them hear what the spirit says to the churches. The victorious one will not be hurt at all by the second death.

Gratitude

Happy 10th birthday to our granddaughter Lainey.

Prayer

For our granddaughter Lainey with her knowledge of Christ and the reality of the Holy Spirit. Bring peace and tranquility to our son Christiaan and his wife Jessica in their move to Elizabethtown. Heal my friend Dale following his surgery.

Today, I will be grateful that my talkative colleague was mostly quiet.

My patient from Africa finished one year of therapy today for HER2-positive locally advanced breast cancer. She is now returning home. She gave me a thank-you card. We had a remarkable meeting of the Susquehanna STEM to the Skies board of directors. The board had multiple helpful suggestions, including a partner-in-command event and school visits to discuss our STEM program later in the year.

Day 87, Psalm 119: 31-32

I hold fast to your statutes, Lord; do not let me be put to shame. I run in the path of your commands, for you have broadened my understanding.

Gratitude

I am grateful that I have a home, children, grandchildren, a profession, and an avocation. I am thankful that an unexpected and significant debt is not financially ruinous to Sally and me.

Prayer

Give us wisdom and clarity of thought to resolve our financial challenge.

Today, I will trust the Lord to guide us.

I learned from Sally that we owe a substantial debt due to the mismanagement of a restoration project. We have maxed our credit cards and our line of credit. We are working with the bank to restructure the debt.

God appeared to show me how to love others when they do something entirely thoughtless and irresponsible.

Day 88, Romans 2: 4

Or do you show contempt for the riches of his kindness, forbearance, and patience, not realizing that God's kindness is intended to lead you to repentance?

Gratitude

Thank you for our weekly men's Bible study, for beautiful flying weather, for a light clinic schedule that allows me to go to the bank in mid-day, and for Heather Buttorff, our banker.

Prayer

For healing of a friend after back surgery, and for Sally and our debt.

Today, I will not show contempt for the richness of God's kindness to me.

We went to the bank, where I learned we now have a new 15-year mortgage to manage our debt crisis at age 69. I flew Russ Stankiewicz to Lancaster Airport to retrieve his plane after his annual inspection. I had a beautiful evening flight home to Selinsgrove just before twilight.

Day 89, Proverbs 1: 8-9

Listen, my son, to your father's instruction and do not forsake your mother's teaching. They are a garland to grace your head in a chain to adorn your neck.

(There were no other entries for this day.)

Day 90, Colossians 1: 13-14

For he has rescued us from the dominion of darkness and brought us into the Kingdom of the son he loves, in whom we have redemption, the forgiveness of sins.

Gratitude

We bought a beautiful hanging flower basket at Davies Market and got lunch at Chipotle. We ate in the boardroom at Penn Valley Airport.

Prayer

Thank you for guiding me to grace and peace over the poor decision-making of a loved one.

Today, I will not punish someone for making very poor financial decisions.

I took Sally to the Redbird FMX simulator at her request and showed her how it operates. We flew a simulated flight from Selinsgrove to Bloomsburg, simulated an engine emergency, and crashed short of Runway 27. We did not yell at each other, violating the rule that a flight instructor should not teach a spouse.

God appeared today in the love and understanding of two spouses.

POSTSCRIPT

Susquehanna STEM to the Skies is a 501(c)(3) public charity that seeks to develop STEM (Science, Technology, Engineering, and Mathematics) educational opportunities in our local schools with an aviation foundation to help broaden school-based STEM education.

The principles of the program are:

Innovation: Our program uses an aviation foundation to introduce STEM skills and inform students and their parents about employment opportunities in multiple aviation-related careers.

Value: Our program provides a simulated or actual flying experience, allowing students to enjoy safely flying an aircraft in a full-motion aviation simulator under the guidance of a certified flight instructor (CFI).

Academics: CFIs introduce and demonstrate STEM concepts, and students get work problem assignments to complete on-site that employ STEM concepts in solving aviation-related tasks.

Susquehanna STEM to the Skies became a 501(c)(3) in December 2020. The calendar year 2021 was a "lost year" due to the COVID-19 pandemic. We spent the year recruiting board members and building relationships with the educational community. By spring 2022, we initiated our academic program, including outreach to middle and high schools, career technical centers, home and cyber school groups, and Scouting organizations. Our focus is on career readiness within the aviation industry (pilots, air traffic controllers, airport managers, mechanics, airline dispatchers, Life Flight crews, military aviation, and drone pilots.)

In May 2022, the Penn Valley Airport hosted 24 Boy and Girl Scouts on a tour of the airport, rotating through six career and STEM stations. All scouts fulfilled the requirements for their Scout Aviation Merit Badge after a full and rewarding seven-hour day. The scouts heard from instructors about aviation careers, preflight, flight planning, and aerodynamics, and all 24 scouts flew at the controls of the Redbird FMX simulator. The airport also holds Open Houses each June so the public can learn about airplane and helicopter transport, maintenance careers, and training pathways.

In partnership with SUN Area Technical Institute, New Berlin, PA, Susquehanna STEM to the Skies offered an after-school STEM Aviation Camp consisting of eight after-school sessions from mid-October to mid-November 2022 to recruit and train students for welding and machining technical careers. Susquehanna STEM to the Skies recruited 24 7th through 9th grade students who attended four after-school welding and machining classes.

Based on its long-standing and ongoing educational successes, Susquehanna STEM to the Skies received $25,600 in educational grants in August 2024. An unrestricted $15,000 grant from the Vanguard Charitable Endowment and a $10,600 grant from the 1994 Degenstein Foundation will allow the program to extend its educational opportunities to additional students at the airport and in their classrooms.

The program continues to be free of charge and includes flights in a full-motion Redbird FMX aviation simulator at the airport. Its success is an answer to the prayers of many individuals.

Further information is available at *www.stemtoskies.org*.

REFERENCES

Kairos: The right moment or occasion. (2020, June 30). Institute for Advanced Study. *https://www.ias.edu/ideas/baert-kairos*

www.ingramcontent.com/pod-product-compliance
Lightning Source LLC
Chambersburg PA
CBHW031448120626
46545CB00006B/2609